The Cholesterol
Counter

The Cholesterol Counter

ISABEL WINCKLER

Arlington Books
Clifford Street, Mayfair
London

THE CHOLESTEROL COUNTER

first published 1978 by
Arlington Books (Publishers) Ltd.,
3 Clifford Street, Mayfair
London, W.1.

© *Isabel Winckler 1978*

Printed in England by
Chapel River Press
Andover, Hampshire

ISBN 85140 281 X

Contents

DIET AND HEALTH

Nutrition is the basis of life, yet few of us pause to examine our diet. We eat because we are hungry, because we enjoy food, or, sometimes, simply because the food is there to be eaten. If we are worried about our weight we may watch our Calorie intake, but, apart from that, pay little attention to the nutritional quality of our diet or to its suitability for our own particular way of life. Faulty nutrition is known to affect general health in many ways. The dramatic effects of undernutrition and dietary deficiency demand attention, the results of over-eating are glaringly obvious, but the importance of the more subtle results of specific dietary excesses is only just beginning to be recognised.

Many of the foods we eat today have been eaten for generations without apparent harm. Our ancestors, however, ate far less highly refined foods and few of them consumed the richer foods in anything like the quantities which are eaten today. Life styles too were very different. Before the invention of the slow combustion engine, walking was the usual method of getting from place to place. There were few mechanical aids either at work or at home. In other words diet was simpler and life less sedentary. We can not turn back the clock, even if we wish to do so, but we can look at our way of life, particularly at our diet, and consider whether it might be worth while making some changes which could improve our general health and, perhaps, reduce the risk of serious illness.

There is a growing amount of evidence which suggests that, under modern living conditions, some of the nutrients contained in common foods may contribute to the development of ill-health if eaten in large amounts and that we could improve our well-being by taking more trouble over our diet. Definite proof is difficult to come by but observations and population studies, made all over the world, suggest that the amount and type of fat we eat, together with the cholesterol content of our diet, contribute significantly to our chances of developing certain types of heart disease.

THE MODERN SCOURGE

The gradual expansion of our knowledge, particularly in the fields of medicine, hygiene and nutrition, has led to an increase in the number of years the average individual may expect to live. In the present century great strides have been made in medicine, surgery and drug development. Many killing diseases, such as tuberculosis, have been virtually conquered and the death rates from others (e.g. pneumonia) dramatically reduced. Yet if we look at the 25 years, 1945-69, we find that there was no significant change in the life-expectancy of men aged 45. Statistics show that 29% of all men die between the ages of 40 and 64. Such figures suggest that while conditions of life generally are improving, and medical science is able to control more and more diseases, some other aspect of life is deteriorating.

Diseases of the heart and blood vessels (cardiovascular diseases) have become the greatest killers of modern times. They are responsible for about half the deaths in England and Wales. Before the last war, coronary heart disease was mainly confined to the rich: now it affects all income groups. In 1973, in Great Britain, 2 of every 5 men who died between the ages of 45 and 54 died of coronary heart disease. In younger men (aged 35-44) about one-third of deaths were from this cause. Women are not immune. After the age of 55 they appear to be just as much at risk as men.

In the United States of America the risk is even higher, but, in Norway, a country containing a large rural population, the incidence is lower than in Britain, while in Asia and Africa it is very low indeed. Cardiovascular disease in general, and coronary heart disease in particular, appear to be diseases of civilisation and urbanisation. It should, therefore, be possible to reduce the risk of developing these conditions by examining the differences in life styles and making any changes that are appropriate and reasonable.

THE CARDIOVASCULAR SYSTEM

The heart, arteries, veins and smaller blood vessels (capillaries) form the transport system of the body. This carries vital oxygen and nutrients to all body tissues and removes harmful waste products. It conveys enzymes and hormones to the places where they are needed to carry out important functions. It transports protective factors to areas where they may be required to help combat infections. Anything that affects the efficiency of this system must have a deleterious effect on health. Anything which seriously blocks the system, preventing the delivery of oxygen and nutrients to body tissues, must have serious consequencies.

The heart is a very efficient muscular pump which

maintains the circulation of the blood within the blood vessels. There are three distinct blood circuits:-

The General Circulation which carries blood to all parts of the body
The Lung Circulation which carries blood to the lungs to be cleared of carbon dioxide and enriched with oxygen
The Heart Circulation, the coronary arteries, which supply the heart muscles themselves with essential oxygen and nutrients.

HOW HEART DISEASE CAN DEVELOP

Healthy blood vessels are lined with very smooth tissue, over which the blood flows easily, but this layer can become thickened and distorted by tiny plates made up of fibrous tissue, fatty substances and blood clots. This condition is known as atherosclerosis. If the damage becomes extensive it results in significant narrowing of the blood vessels. Blood flow is impeded in much the same way as parked cars cause a traffic-jam in a busy street. Normally small blood vessels can relieve the congestion through by-passing the obstruction and carrying the blood to its destination, but if these are also blocked blood supply is shut off from body tissues, depriving them of oxygen. Without oxygen, tissues cease to function and die.

The seriousness of the results of such damage depends on where the blockage occurs. Blockage of the coronary arteries supplying the heart muscles (coronary thrombosis) will damage the heart and result in coronary heart disease. Since this condition is very grave indeed, anything that could prevent or slow up the development of atherosclerosis must be worth trying.

In the past medical care has been aimed mainly at dealing with illness where it occurs. If we could attack the factors likely to cause disease long before it actually develops we could improve our health and lengthen our life span. Almost all individuals in Western Europe and the United States of America have some degree of atherosclerosis, but this condition is much less common in more primitive communities. This appears to be one field where prevention could be easier than cure.

THE DEVELOPMENT OF ATHEROSCLEROSIS

No one factor can be said to cause atherosclerosis. Many widely different by interrelated circumstances seem to contribute to its development. These include:-

Genetic Factors
Stress
Heavy Smoking
Excessive Alcohol Consumption
Lack of Exercise
Diet

GENETIC FACTORS

A small percentage of people never develop atherosclerosis, although they are exposed to the same factors which cause the condition in their neighbours. This appears to be a, so far, unexplained metabolic difference, rather like the unknown factor which enables some people to remain slim while on a high Calorie diet.

On the other hand, some families appear to be particularly liable to develop atherosclerosis. There is nothing we can do about our genetic inheritance but, if we know that there is a familial tendency, we could take particular care not to subject ourselves to the other factors involved in its development.

STRESS

Atherosclerosis is less frequently found in people living and working in rural surroundings. This suggests that exposure to the pace, noise and tension of modern life increases the risk of developing this condition. It is not easy to change our jobs and it is usually impossible to relax or stop worrying to order. Regular exercise can be helpful but the best way to minimise risk is to eliminate other contributory causes.

SMOKING

The heavy increase in cigarette smoking that followed the last war parallels the rise in the incidence of coronary heart disease. There is a lot of evidence to suggest that, in Western countries at least, excessive smoking does increase the risk of developing atherosclerosis.

ALCOHOL

The relationship between heavy drinking and atherosclerosis is not so clearly defined. It is known that a combination of a large amount of alcohol and a rich meal does raise the fat and cholesterol level of the blood. It might be wise if such meals were avoided by executives already subjected to stress.

EXERCISE

Man should be a working animal. Our ancestors obtained all the energy for the work they did from the food they ate. We rely much more on non-human energy, machines at work, machines in the home and mechanical transport. We tend to get our recreation from watching other people expending their energy. This is an unnatural way of life and appears to contribute significantly to the risk of atherosclerosis.

DIET

The blood of people with atherosclerosis always contains high levels of fat and cholesterol. Reduction of these levels is known to reduce the risk of coronary heart disease by 40%. There are 4 ways in which diet may affect these high fat and cholesterol levels:-

Overeating
Type of carbohydrate eaten
Quantity and type of fat eaten
Cholesterol level of diet

Overeating

Carbohydrates and fats, eaten in amounts in excess of each individual's energy needs, are stored as body fat, leading first to overweight and then to obesity, the most common nutritional disease of the Western World. Excess weight is uncomfortable, but obesity is dangerous and much more difficult to correct. Obese people are much more likely to develop bronchitis, arthritis, diabetes and heart disease. The records of life insurance companies show that the life expectancy of a man aged 45 years is decreased by 45% if his weight is 25% above average.

Overeating and lack of exercise are interrelated, creating a vicious circle which it is difficult to break. Underactivity contributes to the development of excess weight and obesity prevents activity. Reduction of body weight is known to lower blood fat and cholesterol levels, thus slowing down the progress of atherosclerosis and lessening the risk of coronary heart disease. So the first dietary step towards the prevention of coronary heart disease must be adjustment of the Calorie content of the diet to the level necessary to achieve and maintain ideal body weight.

The Carbohydrate Content of the Diet

Carbohydrates are eaten in large quantities all over the world. This has always been so because carbohydrates are the cheapest form of energy and form the basis of the great majority of diets. In Britain we rely mainly on wheat and potatoes to supply our carbohydrates. Other countries use wheat in a different form (e.g. as pasta in Italy) or alternative cereals, such as rice. Yet others utilise root vegetables. In all these foods starch is the main carbohydrate present.

In recent years there has been a tendency, by the richer nations, to replace starch by sugar. In fact the great rise in sugar consumption in the United Kingdom is one of the most outstanding dietary changes of the 20th century.

Scientists have pointed out that the rise in sugar consumption parallels the increase in the incidence of coronary heart disease. Studies have also shown that Zulus, whose diet contains about 6 lb sugar per head, per year, have a low incidence of coronary heart disease, while in American negroes, who eat, on average, 80 lb sugar per head, per year, it is quite common. Indians living in Natal, with an average yearly intake of 110 lb sugar have a higher incidence of coronary heart disease than Indians living in India, who eat only about 12 lb per head, per year.

This evidence is not conclusive since diets containing large amounts of sugar are usually richer in other ways. However, it might be prudent to replace some of the sugar we are eating with starch, by eating more bread and potatoes and less cakes, puddings and biscuits. If we do have a weight

page 17

problem, decreasing the amount of sugar-rich foods we eat is an excellent way of dealing with it.

The Fat Content of the Diet

The total quantity of fat in the diet seems to have a very definite effect on the development of atherosclerosis. The plates which are obstructing the blood vessels contain large amounts of fatty materials and blood clots. It is known that meals containing high levels of fat accelerate blood clotting. People whose diets contain a great deal of fat generally have high levels of fat and cholesterol in their blood. Populations of countries where diets contain less fat and patients who are on low-fat diets have much lower levels of both fat and cholesterol in their blood.

In Great Britain our total fat intake is rising. In 1948 we obtained about 33% of our Calories from fat, by 1969 this had risen to 42%. Reduction of total fat intake could lead to lowering of blood fat and cholesterol levels and reduced risk of development of coronary heart disease.

It is, however, not only the total amount of fat we eat that is important but also the type. Our diet contains both animal fats and vegetable oils (which are simply fats which normally remain liquid at room temperature). Fats and oils are composed of glycerol (an alcohol) and fatty acids. Each unit of glycerol can combine with 3 fatty acid units and all oils and fats contain a mixture of these acids.

There are two main types of fatty acids.

Saturated which are found mainly in animal products (fat meat, milk, eggs, etc.). Fats composed mainly of saturated fatty acids are usually solid at room temperature.

Unsaturated which are found mainly in vegetable oils and in fish. Fats composed mainly of unsaturated fatty acids are usually liquid at room temperature.

Experiments have shown that when saturated fats are eaten blood cholesterol levels are raised, while unsaturated fats tend to lower these levels.

Many doctors believe that substitution of part of our normal intake of animal fat with vegetable oil could help to reduce the incidence of coronary heart disease.

Cholesterol in the Diet

Cholesterol is a fatty substance which derives its name from the Greek words chole (bile) and steros (solid).

Over 60 years ago a report was published which

showed that diets high in cholesterol and saturated fats raise levels of both cholesterol and fat in the blood. Since that time many more studies have been published and over 100 of these confirm the original report.

It is more difficult to assess the importance of dietary cholesterol because this substance is found in all healthy individuals and is actually produced by the liver in our own bodies. It is an ingredient of bile salts, which are essential for the digestion of fat, and it is always present in healthy blood, where it helps to transport fatty acids.

Nevertheless, the amount of cholesterol in our food does affect the level of cholesterol in our blood. Nations like the Japanese who eat a diet containing low levels of cholesterol have low blood levels. People in Northern Europe and the United States of America generally have high levels of cholesterol in their diet which are matched by their blood levels. If the level of cholesterol in the diet is low, little of it is absorbed by the digestive system, but, at high dietary levels, a greater proportion is absorbed.

In no race with habitually high cholesterol intakes is atherosclerosis absent. If intake is low this condition is not prevalent. Risk of the development of coronary heart disease rises with the level of cholesterol in the blood. It has been claimed that men with a blood cholesterol level of 280 mg per 100 ml are 4 times as likely to have a heart attack as men with levels below 200 mg per 100 ml.

Of the many factors which contribute to the development of atherosclerosis and coronary heart disease, heavy smoking, lack of exercise and bad dietary habits could be avoided. The development of a new eating plan could be most rewarding since not only could it help us improve our own health, but, by changing family meals we would bring up our children on a safer diet and, perhaps, help to create a generation relatively free from atherosclerosis.

As long ago as 1964 the American Heart Association considered that there was sufficient evidence to justify the publication of a statement advising the public to make dietary modifications. Following this advice the Anti-Coronary Club, based in New York, sponsored a study in which 814 healthy men, aged between 40 and 54 years, ate a diet low in saturated fats and cholesterol for 7 years. Not only were their blood cholesterol levels shown to be lower than those of a similar group of 436 men eating the normal American diet, but they also had a significantly lower incidence of coronary heart disease.

The Combined Medical Boards of Norway, Sweden and Finland have a definite policy in encouraging the reduction of total fat and the replacement of some saturated fat with unsaturated fat, any decrease in Calories to be made up with starch, not sugar. Recommendations have also been made by many doctors in the Netherlands, Germany, Australia and the United Kingdom.

RULES FOR HEALTHIER EATING

Adjust Calorie intake to the level required to reach and maintain ideal body weight.
Do not eat too much sugar or sweet foods.
Reduce total fat intake to a level which will supply no more than 25-30% of total Calories.
Replace part of saturated fat content of diet with unsaturated fat.
Reduce cholesterol intake to 300 mg per day.

HOW TO ACHIEVE A HEALTHIER DIET

CALORIE RESTRICTION
If the weight problem is slight, reduction in total

fat intake may be enough to correct it. Giving up sugar and eating less sweet foods will also help. If you need advice consult Jane Colin's *Pocket Calorie Guide to Safer Slimming*.

TOTAL FAT REDUCTION

The amount of fat your diet should contain will depend on your Calorie needs.

TABLE 1

Calorie Allowance	Fat Allowance
1000	27-32 g
1500	40-48 g
2000	54-65 g
2500	67-81 g

Remember that, besides the visible fats (butter, margarine, lard, oil, cream, and fat meats) there are a lot of invisible fats in such foods as cheese, eggs, cakes, puddings and biscuits.

The Tables on pages 32-41 will help you to replan your diet.

MODIFICATION OF FAT INTAKE

This simply means substituting vegetable oils for some of the hard fats you eat and using fish in place of some animal products.

FOODS CONTAINING SATURATED FATS

TABLE 2

Foods Containing Saturated Fats

Milk (except skimmed)	Bacon
Cream	Fat Meat
Icecream	Sausages
Butter	Cakes, Puddings, Pastry
*Hard Margarine	Biscuits
Lard	Lemon Curd
Cooking Fat	Toffees
Dripping	Mincemeat

FOODS CONTAINING UNSATURATED FATS

TABLE 3

Foods Containing Unsaturated Fats

Vegetable Oils	Herring
*Soft Margarines	Kippers
Salmon	Mackerel

* Although margarine is made from oil, many brands are hardened by a process known as hydrogenation, which converts some of the unsaturated fatty acids to saturated fatty acids. The magarines which contain the highest

proportion of unsaturated fatty acids are those whose consistency is like that of whipped cream (e.g. Flora).

Substitution is not difficult if you follow a few simple rules.

Cut off all visible fat from meat.

Use oil for frying, grilling and roasting, instead of lard, cooking fat or dripping.

Use soft margarine on bread and for making pastry, cakes and biscuits.

Use low-fat cheeses, i.e. cottage instead of cream and Edam instead of Cheddar.

Do not make gravy from the drip in the roasting pan.

Avoid rich sauces.

Examine the labels on processed foods. Vegetable oils are unsaturated, animal fats and hydrogenated vegetable oils are saturated.

CHOLESTEROL RESTRICTION

Keeping your eye on the cholesterol content of your diet is more difficult than counting Calories because comprehensive tables are not yet available.

Cholesterol is found only in products of animal origin. Levels are higher in young than in older animals so there will be more in veal and lamb than in beef and mutton. Although cholesterol is a fatty substance it does attach itself to protein, so will be found in lean as well as fat meat. The highest meat sources are brain and offal.

In general cholesterol levels are slightly lower in fish than in meat and it is mainly concentrated in the skin, oil and liver.

Egg yolk is a very high course indeed but there is no cholesterol in egg white.

The tables on pages 42-53, taken from figures published by the United States Department of Agriculture, will help you to keep the cholesterol level of your diet below the recommended level.

DIETARY CARE

To remain healthy we need adequate supplies of a wide range of nutrients. Any dietary restriction is unwise unless we take care to rebalance our diet. It is so easy to give in to the temptation to achieve our ends by living on a limited selection of foods, but we are aiming at HEALTHIER EATING. This demands a good mixed diet.

ENERGY

If there is no weight problem, the Calories lost by reducing fat intake should be made up by eating more carbohydrate, choosing foods containing starch (bread, potatoes, rice, pasta) rather than those containing large amounts of sugar.

PROTEIN

Protein is essential, not only for growth in children, but also to adults for repair and renewal of body tissues and to help guard against infections. Meat, fish and eggs are the best sources. Use as much animal protein as you can within your cholesterol allowance and make up with:

TABLE 4

Wheat Germ	Bread
Nuts	Beans and Lentils
Oatmeal	Semolina

VITAMIN B

This is a group name for a number of vitamins which are essential for the conversion of carbohydrate to energy. Two of these vitamins, riboflavin and niacin, could be in short supply in your changed diet.

Riboflavin is normally mainly supplied from milk and its products. Milk is a good food and should not be left out. You can reduce its saturated fat and cholesterol content by using skim (either liquid or powdered). Niacin is mainly provided by meat. See that your diet contains:

TABLE 5

Wheat Germ	Nuts
Dried Fruit	Beans
Oatmeal	Low-fat Yoghurt

CALCIUM

This mineral is essential throughout life to maintain bone structure. It is mainly supplied by milk and cheese. Make up with:

TABLE 6

Cottage Cheese	Green Vegetables
Low-fat Yoghurt	Almonds
Bread	

IRON

Iron is essential for healthy blood and, if the diet does not contain sufficient, one type of anaemia is likely to develop. The main sources of this mineral are meat, particularly offal. Other valuable sources are:

TABLE 7

| Wheat Germ | Green Vegetables |
| Bread | Dried Fruit |

The meals on pages 62-69 will help you to start planning your diet. Get to know more about foods, the more you know the easier it will be for you to choose the right type of food for your new, healthier diet.

HOW TO USE THE TABLES

THE FAT CONTENT OF SOME COMMON FOODS

Use these tables to ensure that fat is providing no more than 25-30% of your total Calorie intake (see page 13). You will see that many innocent foods, such as chocolate cake, contribute quite large amounts of fat to your diet. Read through the tables and note the main pit-falls.

Three sets of figures are given in the tables.

mg/oz — milligrammes of fat present in one ounce of food, ready to eat.

mg/100 g — milligrammes of fat present in 100 grammes of food, ready to eat.

Average Helping — milligrammes of fat present in an average portion. Peoples' ideas of average helpings vary a great deal, but the accompanying notes will help you.

CHOLESTEROL COUNTER

Use these tables to estimate the amount of cholesterol your diet contains and try to keep your daily intake below 300 mg.

Three sets of figures are given.

mg/oz — milligrammes of cholesterol present in one ounce of food, ready to eat.

mg/100 g — milligrammes of cholesterol present in 100 grammes of food, ready to eat.

Average Helping — milligrammes of cholesterol present in an average portion. These helpings are the same size as those in the fat tables, to help you plan your meals easily.

THE FAT CONTENT OF SOME COMMON FOODS

Dairy Products and Fats	g/oz	g/100g
Butter	24.2	85.1
Cheese, Cheddar	9.8	34.5
Cheese, cream	24.5	86.0
Cheese, cottage	0.15	0.5
Cheese, Edam	6.5	22.9
Cooking oil	28.3	99.9
Cream, double	13.7	48.2
Cream, single	6.0	21.2
Egg	3.5	12.3
Lard	28.1	99.0
Margarine	24.2	85.3
Milk, whole	1.1	3.7
Milk, skim	0.1	0.2
Milk, canned condensed (sweetened)	3.4	12.0
Milk, canned evaporated (unsweetened)	2.4	8.4
Outline	11.3	39.6
Suet	28.1	99.0

Dairy Products and Fats	Average Helping	g
Butter	1 Tablespoon	12.0
Cheese, Cheddar	1 oz	9.8
Cheese, cream	1 Tablespoon	12.0
Cheese, cottage	1 cup	1.3
Cheese, Edam	1 oz	6.5
Cooking oil	1 Tablespoon	14.0
Cream, double	1 Tablespoon	7.2
Cream, single	1 Tablespoon	3.2
Egg	1 large	6.2
Lard	1 Tablespoon	13.9
Margarine	1 Tablespoon	11.9
Milk, whole	1 cup	9.0
Milk, skim	1 cup	0.5
Milk, canned condensed (sweetened)	1 cup	36.7
Milk, canned evaporated (unsweetened)	1 cup	21.2
Outline	1 Tablespoon	5.5
Suet	1 oz	28.1

Meat, Poultry and Game	g/oz	g/100g
Bacon, fried (average)	12.0	42.0
Beef, roast	9.1	32.1
Beef steak, grilled	6.1	21.6
Chicken, roast	2.1	7.3
Duck, roast	6.7	23.6
Ham, boiled	11.2	39.6
Lamb, roast	5.6	20.4
Liver, fried	4.1	14.5
Luncheon meat	7.8	29.0
Pork, roast	11.5	40.4
Sausage, beef, fried	5.2	18.4
Sausage, pork, fried	7.1	24.8
Sausage, breakfast	5.8	20.4
Tongue	6.8	23.9
Turkey, roast	2.2	7.7
Veal cutlet, fried	2.3	8.1

Meat, Poultry and Game	Average Helping	g
Bacon, fried (average)	2 thin rashers, 8″ long	6.7
Beef, roast	4 thin slices, 4⅛″ x 2¼″	27.3
Beef steak, grilled	3 oz	18.3
Chicken, roast	3 slices, 3½″ x 2½″	6.6
Duck, roast	3 slices, 3½″ x 2½″	23.6
Ham, boiled	1 slice, 5″ x 4½″ x ⅛″	17.8
Lamb, roast	1 slice, 4½″ x 3½″ x ⅛″	10.2
Liver, fried	1 piece, 3″ x 3″ x ¾″	14.5
Luncheon meat	1 slice, 4″ x 4″ x ⅛″	9.0
Pork, roast	1 slice, 3″ x 2½″ x ¼″	24.2
Sausage, beef, fried	1	6.1
Sausage, pork, fried	1	8.2
Sausage, breakfast	1 slice, 4½″ dia. ⅛″ thick	6.3
Tongue	4 slices, 3″ x 2″ x ⅛″	9.1
Turkey, roast	1 slice, 4″ x 2½″ x ¼″	3.9
Veal cutlet, fried	1	13.0

Fish and Shellfish	g/oz	g/100g
Cod, fried	1.3	4.7
Crab, boiled	1.5	5.2
Eels, stewed	9.2	32.2
Haddock, fried	2.4	8.3
Hake, fried	3.2	11.4
Herring, grilled	4.3	15.1
Kipper, baked	3.2	11.1
Mackerel, fried	3.2	11.1
Pilchard, canned	3.1	10.8
Plaice, fried	4.1	14.4
Salmon, fresh, boiled	3.7	13.0
Salmon, canned	1.7	6.0
Sardine, canned	6.4	22.6
Spratt, smoked, grilled	6.6	23.2
Trout, steamed	1.3	4.5

Cereals, Cakes, Puddings, etc.	Average Helping	g
Apple pie	⅛th 9″ dia. pie	8.9
Biscuits, plain, mixed	3	2.4
Biscuits, sweet, mixed	3	3.7
Bread, fried	1 small slice	11.2
Cherry cake	1/16th 9″ dia. cake	18.0
Chocolate cake	1/16th 9″ dia. cake	19.0
Coconut cake	1/16th 9″ dia. cake	18.5

Fish and Shellfish	Average Helping	g
Cod, fried	Steak, 3½" x 2½" x 1"	5.4
Crab, boiled	1 cup	6.5
Eels, stewed	4 oz	36.8
Haddock, fried	Piece, 4" x 3" x ½"	8.3
Hake, fried	Piece, 4" x 3" x ½"	11.4
Herring, grilled	1 small	15.1
Kipper, baked	1 small	11.1
Mackerel, fried	Fillet, 8½" x 2½" x ½"	11.7
Pilchard, canned	3 oz	9.3
Plaice, fried	4 oz	16.4
Salmon, fresh, boiled	Piece, 6¾" x 2½" x 1"	18.9
Salmon, canned	½ cup	4.5
Sardine, canned	4, 3" long	10.6
Spratt, smoked, grilled	8, 3" long	21.8
Trout, steamed	4 oz	5.2

Cereals, Cakes, Puddings, etc.	g/oz	g/100g
Apple pie	2.1	7.5
Biscuits, plain mixed	3.8	13.2
Biscuits, sweet mixed	8.7	30.7
Bread, fried	10.6	37.2
Cherry cake	6.8	24.0
Chocolate cake	7.2	25.4
Coconut cake	7.0	24.6

Cereals, Cakes,
Puddings, etc. (cont.)

	g/oz	g/100g
Doughnut	4.5	15.8
Dundee cake	4.3	15.0
Eccles cake	8.9	31.6
Gingerbread	3.7	13.0
Jam roll	5.4	19.0
Jam tart	4.4	15.4
Lemon curd tart	7.1	25.0
Mince pie	6.3	22.3
Pancake	4.3	15.1
Pastry, flaky	11.9	42.0
Pastry, short	9.5	33.4
Queen cake	6.4	22.5
Rock cake	4.5	16.0
Scone	3.7	13.2
Shortbread	7.7	27.2
Suet pudding	5.6	19.8
Syrup sponge	4.4	15.4
Trifle	1.6	5.6
Victoria sandwich	7.2	25.3
Wheat germ	2.6	9.3
Yorkshire pudding	2.7	9.4

Cereals, Cakes,

Puddings, etc. (cont.)	*Average Helping* ·	*g*
Doughnut	1	5.1
Dundee cake	1/16th 9″ dia. cake	14.3
Eccles cake	1	17.8
Gingerbread	1/9 8″ square	8.2
Jam roll	1 slice, 1″ x 2″ dia.	10.8
Jam tart	1 small	6.6
Lemon curd tart	1 small	10.6
Mince pie	1 small	12.6
Pancake	1, 6″ dia.	
	(7 tablespoons batter)	11.0
Pastry, flaky	1 oz	11.9
Pastry, short	1 oz	9.5
Queen cake	1 small	9.6
Rock cake	1 small	9.0
Scone	1 small	5.6
Shortbread	1, 2″ x ¾″	3.8
Suet pudding	1 cup	22.4
Syrup sponge	1 cup	13.2
Trifle	1 cup	3.2
Victoria sandwich	1/16th 9″ dia.	19.0
Wheat germ	1 oz	2.6
Yorkshire pudding	1, 3″ dia.	6.8

Vegetables, Fruits _and Nuts_	g/oz	g/100g
Almonds	15.2	53.5
Avocado pear	2.3	8.0
Brazil nuts	17.3	61.5
Cob nuts	10.2	36.0
Coconut, dessicated	17.6	62.0
Mushrooms, fried	6.4	22.3
Onions, fried	9.5	33.3
Peanuts	13.9	49.0
Potato, chips	2.6	9.0
Potato, crisps	10.2	39.6
Tomato, fried	1.7	5.9
Walnuts	14.6	51.5

Sauces, Preserves _and Sweets_		
Cheese sauce	3.7	13.0
Chocolate (average)	10.4	36.4
Cocoa powder	6.6	25.6
Custard sauce	1.1	3.9
Ice cream	3.2	11.3
Lemon curd	3.9	13.9
Salad cream	10.2	36.0
White sauce	2.8	9.7

Vegetables, Fruits and Nuts	Average Helping	g
Almonds	10	7.0
Avocado pear	½, 3″ long	8.0
Brazil nuts	10	39.4
Cob nuts	10	5.4
Coconut, dessicated	¼ cup	9.9
Mushrooms, fried	5	11.2
Onions, fried	½ cup	35.0
Peanuts	20	8.8
Potato, chips	16	7.2
Potato, crisps	1 oz	10.2
Tomato, fried	2 medium	8.9
Walnuts	12 halves	7.7

Sauces, Preserves and Sweets	Average Helping	
Cheese sauce	1 cup	32.5
Chocolate (average)	1 oz	10.4
Cocoa powder	2 teaspoonfuls	1.8
Custard sauce	1 cup	9.8
Ice cream	1 cup	15.0
Lemon curd	1 Tablespoonful	2.8
Salad cream	1 Tablespoonful	5.0
White sauce	1 cup	24.3

THE CHOLESTEROL COUNTER

Dairy Products and Fats	mg/oz	mg/100g
Butter	71	250
Buttermilk	0.6	2
Cheese, blue	25	87
Cheese, Camembert	26	92
Cheese, Cheddar	28	99
Cheese, cottage	3	9
Cheese, cream	32	111
Cheese, Edam	29	102
Cheese, Limburger	28	98
Cheese, Mozzarella	28	97
Cheese, Meunster	26	91
Cheese, Neufchatel	22	76
Cheese, Parmesan	32	113
Cheese, Swiss	30	100
Cheese, processed, American	26	90
Cheese, processed, Swiss	26	93
Cheese spread	18	64
Cheese souffle	47	167
Cheese straws	9	32
Cooking oil	0	0
Cream, double	38	133
Cream, single	19	66
Cream, sour	19	66

Dairy Products and Fats	Average Helping	mg
Butter	1 Tablespoonful	35
Buttermilk	1 cup	5
Cheese, blue	1 oz	25
Cheese, Camembert	Section $2\frac{3}{8}''$ x $2\frac{1}{4}''$ x $1''$	39
Cheese, Cheddar	1 oz	28
Cheese, cottage	1 cup	23
Cheese, cream	1 Tablespoonful	16
Cheese, Edam	1 oz	29
Cheese, Limburger	1 oz	28
Cheese, Mozzarella	1 oz	28
Cheese, Meunster	1 oz	26
Cheese, Neufchatel	1 oz	22
Cheese, Parmesan	1 cup, grated	113
Cheese, Swiss	Slice, $7\frac{1}{2}''$ x $4''$ x $\frac{1}{16}''$	35
Cheese, processed, American	Slice, $3\frac{1}{2}''$ x $3\frac{3}{8}''$ x $\frac{1}{8}''$	25
Cheese, processed, Swiss	Slice, $3\frac{1}{2}''$ x $3\frac{3}{8}''$ x $\frac{1}{8}''$	26
Cheese spread	1 Tablespoonful	9
Cheese souffle	1 cup	184
Cheese straws	10 pieces, $5''$ x $\frac{3}{8}''$ x $\frac{3}{8}''$	19
Cooking oil		0
Cream, double	1 Tablespoonful	20
Cream, single	1 Tablespoonful	10
Cream, sour	1 Tablespoonful	8

Dairy Products and Fats (cont.)	mg/oz	mg/100g
Egg, boiled	143	504
Egg, scrambled	117	411
Egg, white	0	0
Egg, yolk	420	1480
Lard	27	95
Margarine, containing animal fat (average)	14	50
*Margarine, vegetable oil only	0	0
Milk, whole	4	14
Milk, skim	0.6	2
Milk, canned, condensed (sweetened)	10	34
Milk, canned, evaporated (unsweetened)	9	31
Milk, dried, instant whole	31	109
Milk, dried, instant non-fat	6	22
Outline	0	0
Welsh rarebit	9	31
Yoghurt, low-fat, plain	2	8
Yoghurt, low-fat, fruit	2	7

*Vegetable Oil Margarines:

Alfonal	Flora
Bluexband	Golden Corn
Coop Good Life	Luxury
Coop Luxury	Tomar

Dairy Products and Fats (cont.)	Average Helping	mg
Eggs, boiled	1	252
Eggs, scrambled	1 with milk and fat	263
Egg, white		0
Egg, yolk	1	252
Lard	1 cup	195
Margarine, containing animal fat (average)	1 Tablespoonful	7
Margarine, vegetable oil only		0
Milk, whole	1 cup	34
Milk, skim	1 cup	5
Milk, canned, condensed (sweetened)	1 cup	103
Milk, canned, evaporated (unsweetened)	1 cup	79
Milk, dried, instant whole	1 cup (dry)	75
Milk, dried, instant non-fat	1 cup (dry)	15
Outline		0
Welsh rarebit	1 cup	71
Yoghurt, low-fat, plain	8 oz	17
Yoghurt, low-fat, fruit	8 oz	13

Meat, Poultry and Game	mg/oz	mg/100g
Beef, lean and fat	27	94
Beef, lean only	26	91
Beef and vegetable stew	7	26
Brains	568	2000
Chicken, breast	23	80
Chicken, gizzard	41	145
Chicken, heart	66	231
Chicken, leg	26	91
Chicken liver	212	746
Chicken a la king	22	76
Chicken fricassee	11	40
Chicken and noodles	11	40
Chicken chop suey	7	26
Chicken chow mein	9	31
Heart, beef	78	274
Kidney, beef, calf, lamb and pork	228	804
Lamb, lean and fat	28	98
Lamb, lean only	28	98
Liver, beef, calf, lamb and pork	124	438
Pork, lean and fat	25	89
Pork, lean only	25	89
Sausage, Frankfurter	18	62
Turkey, breast	22	77
Turkey, gizzard	65	229
Turkey, heart	68	238

Meat, Poultry and Game	Average Helping	mg
Beef, lean and fat	4 thin slices, 4⅛" x 2¼"	80
Beef, lean only	4 thin slices, 4⅛" x 2¼"	77
Beef and vegetable stew	1 cup	63
Brains	3 oz	1704
Chicken, breast	½ breast from 3 lb chicken	74
Chicken, gizzard	1 oz	41
Chicken, heart	1 oz	66
Chicken, leg	1 drumstick from 3 lb chicken	47
Chicken, liver	Piece, 2" x 2" x ⅝"	187
Chicken a la king	1 cup	185
Chicken fricassee	1 cup	96
Chicken and noodles	1 cup	96
Chicken chop suey	1 cup	64
Chicken chow mein	1 cup	77
Heart, beef	1 cup (diced)	398
Kidney, beef, calf, lamb and pork	1 cup (slices)	1125
Lamb, lean and fat	4 thin slices, 4⅛" x 2¼"	83
Lamb, lean only	4 thin slices, 4⅛" x 2¼"	83
Liver, beef, calf, lamb and pork	Slice, 6½" x 2⅜" x ⅜"	372
Pork, lean and fat	2 slices, 4⅛" x 2¼" x ¼"	76
Pork, lean only	2 slices, 4⅛" x 2¼" x ¼"	76
Sausage, Frankfurter	1	34

Meat, Poultry and Game (cont.)	mg/oz	mg/100g
Turkey, leg	29	101
Turkey, liver	170	599
Veal, lean and fat	29	101
Veal, lean only	28	99
Rabbit	26	91
Sweetbreads	132	466

*Meat, Poultry
  and Game
  (cont.)*

	Average Helping	
Turkey, breast	2 pieces, 4″ x 2″ x ¼″	65
Turkey, gizzard	1 oz	65
Turkey, heart	1 oz	68
Turkey, leg	4 pieces, 2½″ x 1⅝″ x ¼″	86
Turkey, liver	1 cup (chopped)	839
Veal, lean and fat	3 slices, 2½″ x 2½″	86
Veal, lean only	3 slices, 2½″ x 2½″	84
Rabbit	1 cup (diced)	127
Sweetbreads	2, 3½″ long	536

Fish and Shellfish	mg/oz	mg/100g
Caviar	85	300
Clams	14	50
Clams, canned	18	63
Clam, fritters	37	129
Cod, fresh	14	50
Cod, dried salted	23	82
Crab, fresh	28	100
Crab, canned	29	101
Crab, devilled	29	102
Crab, Imperial	40	140
Flounder	14	50
Haddock	17	60
Halibut	17	60
Herring	24	85
Herring, canned	28	97
Lobster	24	85
Lobster, Newburgh	52	182
Mackerel	29	101
Oysters	14	50
Oysters, canned	13	45
Oyster stew	7	26
Salmon, fresh	13	47
Salmon, canned	10	35
Salmon, roe	102	360
Sardine, canned in oil	40	140
Scallops	15	53
Shrimps	43	150

Fish and Shellfish	Average Helping	mg
Caviar	1 Tablespoon	48
Clams	1 cup	114
Clams, canned	½ cup	50
Clam, fritters	1, 2″ dia.	51
Cod, fresh	Steak, 3½″ x 2½″ x 1″	57
Cod, dried salted	Piece, 5½″ x 1½″ x ½″	66
Crab, fresh	1 cup	125
Crab, canned	1 cup	161
Crab, devilled	1 cup	244
Crab Imperial	1 cup	308
Flounder	Fillet, 4″ x 3″	50
Haddock	Piece, 4″ x 3″ x ½″	60
Halibut	Piece, 6½″ x 2½″ x ⅝″	75
Herring	1 small	85
Herring, canned	1 small	97
Lobster	1 cup	123
Lobster Newburgh	1 cup	456
Mackerel	Fillet, 8½″ x 2½″ x ½″	106
Oysters	1 cup	120
Oysters, canned	½ cup	54
Oyster stew	1 cup	63
Salmon, fresh	Steak, 6¾″ x 2½″ x 1″	59
Salmon, canned	½ cup	26
Salmon, roe	1 oz	102
Sardine, canned in oil	4, 3″ long	66
Scallops	6 medium	78
Shrimps		

Fish and Shellfish (cont.)	mg/oz	mg/100g
Shrimps, canned	43	150
Trout	16	55
Tuna, canned in oil	18	65
Tuna, canned in water	18	63

Fish and Shellfish (cont.)	*Average Helping*	*mg*
Shrimps, canned	1 cup	192
Trout	4 oz	64
Tuna, canned in oil	½ cup	53
Tuna, canned in water	½ cup	51

Although cereals themselves contain no cholesterol, they are rarely eaten alone. They are usually combined with fat, milk or eggs, and may contain these ingredients when purchased. The cholesterol content of cereal foods will depend on the quantity and type of fat they contain together with the proportion of other cholesterol-containing additives.

Cereals, Cakes, Puddings, etc.	mg/oz	mg/100g
Apple pie	0	0
Blancmange	4	14
Bread and Butter pudding	18	64
Chocolate cake	12	43
Custard, baked	30	105
Custard tart	29	105
Fruit cake	13	45
Gingerbread	0.3	1
Ice cream, 10% fat	11	40
Ice cream, 16% fat	16	57
Ice cream, made with eggs	21	73
Lemon chiffon pie	48	169
Lemon meringue pie	25	93
Macaroni cheese	6	21
Muffins	15	53
Noodles, made with eggs	9	31
Pancakes	21	74
Peach pie	0	0
Pumpkin pie	17	61
Rice pudding with raisins	3	11
Spaghetti, with meat balls in tomato sauce	9	30
Sponge cake	70	246
Tapioca pudding	28	97
Waffles	17	60

Cereals, Cakes, Puddings, etc.	Average Helping	mg
Apple pie	⅛ pie 9" dia.	0
Blancmange	1 cup	35
Bread and Butter pudding	1 cup	170
Chocolate cake	$\frac{1}{16}$ cake, 9" dia.	32
Custard, baked	1 cup	278
Custard tart	⅛ tart, 9" dia.	120
Fruit cake	$\frac{1}{30}$, 8" loaf	7
Gingerbread	$\frac{1}{9}$, 8" square	trace
Ice cream (10% fat)	1 cup	53
Ice cream (16% fat)	1 cup	85
Ice cream, made with eggs	1 cup	97
Lemon chiffon pie	⅛ pie, 9" dia.	137
Lemon meringue pie	⅛ pie, 9" dia.	98
Macaroni cheese	1 cup	42
Muffins	1, 3" dia.	21
Noodles, made with eggs	1 cup	50
Pancakes	1, 6" dia.	54
Peach pie		0
Pumpkin pie	⅛ pie, 9" dia.	70
Rice pudding with raisins	1 cup	29
Spaghetti, with meat balls in tomato sauce	1 cup	75
Sponge cake	$\frac{1}{12}$ cake, 10" dia.	162
Tapioca pudding	1 cup	159
Waffles	1, 9" x 9" x ⅝"	119

VEGETABLES AND SAUCES

Although vegetables contain no cholesterol they are often served with butter or sauces which can add quite a lot of cholesterol to the diet.

Vegetables and Sauces	mg/oz	mg/100g
Cheese sauce	5	18
Peppers, stuffed with meat	9	30
Potatoes, au gratin	4	15
Potatoes, scalloped	2	6
Potato salad, with mayonnaise	19	65
Mayonnaise	20	70
Salad dressing	14	50
White sauce, thin	4	14
White sauce, medium	4	13
White sauce, thick	3	12

Vegetables and Sauces	Average Helping	mg
Cheese sauce	1 cup	44
Peppers, stuffed with meat	1, 2¾" x 2½" x 1⅛"	56
Potatoes au gratin	1 cup	36
Potatoes, scalloped	1 cup	14
Potato salad, with mayonnaise	1 cup	162
Mayonnaise	1 Tablespoonful	10
Salad dressing	1 Tablespoonful	8
White sauce, thin	1 cup	64
White sauce, medium	1 cup	59
White sauce, thick	1 cup	55

MEALS FOR HEALTH

Diet has become a depressing word. It suggests restriction, boredom and deprivation. But, if we go back to the dictionary definition of the word — A WAY OF EATING — we can perhaps come to terms with the idea of modifying our own choice of meals to achieve a better diet. Food is part of life, part of living, it must not become a burden but it could be a means of ensuring a healthier way of life.

Our family food habits have developed slowly over the years, it would be a pity to abandon them altogether. It is much better to adapt the recipes the family like to the new scheme.

We all have our own food preferences and these can be retained. If you love meat, have one meat meal a day, restricting the other meals to balance up the day's cholesterol intake. If you mix vegetables with the meat (in stews and pies) you reduce both the cholesterol and the saturated fat content of the meal.

Never let your meals become dull, boredom is the enemy of health. Be adventurous, use the fat and cholesterol tables and experiment.

Your new regime can fit in with family meals. Butter, cream, gravies and sauces can be served separately. Better still get the family involved. The earlier you start the better chance you have of achieving low blood cholesterol levels and reducing the risk of developing coronary heart disease.

REMEMBER
No food is bad if eaten in moderation.
Meals must be attractive. Since you are avoiding rich sauces, use lemon juice or vinegar to give flavour to vegetables and marinade meats in oil with herbs, lemon juice, tomato or wine.
Everyone needs an occasional celebration. If eating out avoid eggs, pate, rich sauces and sweets. You can still have a very enjoyable meal.

Mix and match the following meals to make your own daily plan. They are not all low-cholesterol meals, some contain moderately high levels, but these can be combined with meals with relatively low levels to bring your average daily intake down to the recommended level whilst providing variety in your diet.
The cholesterol and fat content of each meal is given.
U means that the fat in the meal is mainly unsaturated.
S means that the fat in the meal is mainly saturated.

U/S means that the fat in the meal is roughly half unsaturated and half saturated.

NOTE
Skim milk is used in coffee, tea, puddings and other cooked dishes.
Whole milk is used on cereals. If you wish to use skim milk for this purpose you will reduce the cholesterol and saturated fat content of the meal significantly.
Soft vegetable margarine is used on bread and toast.
Cakes, puddings and pastry are home-made, using vegetable margarine as the only form of fat.
Oil is used for frying.
Visible fat is cut off all meat.

Breakfasts

Grapefruit
Toast, margarine and
　　marmalade
Tea or Coffee
　　　Cholesterol 2.5mg
　　　　　Fat 12.5 g (U)

Poached Haddock

Toast and margarine
Tea or Coffee
　　　Cholesterol 62.5 mg
　　　　　Fat 18 g (U)

Kedgeree (no egg)
Toast and margarine
Tea or Coffee
   Cholesterol 32.5 mg
      Fat 15 g (U)

Fresh fruit
Roll and margarine
Tea or Coffee
   Cholesterol 2.5 mg
      Fat 12.5 g (U)

Porridge with milk

Tea or Coffee
   Cholesterol 22.5 mg
      Fat 6 g (S)

Banana, wheat germ and
   milk
Tea or Coffee
   Cholesterol 12.5 mg
      Fat 6 g (U/S)

Bacon (1 rasher) and
   tomatoes
Toast and margarine
Tea or Coffee
   Cholesterol 9.5 mg
      Fat 17 g (U/S)

Meuseli with milk
Tea or Coffee

   Cholesterol 22.5 mg
      Fat 6 g (S)

Orange juice
Toast, margarine and
   marmalade
Tea or Coffee
Cholesterol 2.5 mg
      Fat 12.5 g (U)

Grilled mushrooms on
   toast
Tea or Coffee

   Cholesterol 2.5 mg
      Fat 7 g (U)

Grilled tomatoes on
  toast
Tea or Coffee
    Cholesterol 2.5 mg
        Fat 2 g (U)

Breakfast cereal, wheat
  germ and milk
Tea or Coffee
    Cholesterol 22.5 mg
        Fat 8.5 g (U/S)

Main Meals
Orange juice
Macaroni cheese
Tomatoes
Blackberry and apple
  compote
    Cholesterol 42 mg
        Fat 26 g (S)

Grapefruit
Grilled steak, mush-
  rooms, tomatoes
Potatoes
Apple meringue
    Cholesterol 77 mg
        Fat 22.5 g (S)

Stewed fruit with wheat
germ
Tea or Coffee
    Cholesterol 2.5 mg
        Fat 3 g (U)

Potato cakes and
  tomatoes
Tea or Coffee
    Cholestrol 2.5 mg
        Fat 14.5 g (U)

Lentil soup
Soused herring
Peas, potatoes
Fresh fruit salad

    Cholesterol 85 mg
        Fat 15 g (U)

Tomato and onion salad
Vegetable stew with
  dumplings
Tinned peaches

    Cholesterol 0
        Fat 26 g (U)

Celery soup
Grilled plaice, parsley
    margarine
Carrots, potatoes
Biscuits and cheese
    Cholesterol 86 mg
    Fat 24 g (U/S)

Avocado vinaigrette
Chicken and vegetable
    casserole
Potatoes
Semolina pudding
    Cholesterol 77 mg
    Fat 15 g (U/S)

Tomato Soup
Vegetable curry with
    rice
Mandarin oranges
    Cholesterol 0
    Fat 14 g (U)

Vegetable soup
Fish pie
French beans
Treacle tart
    Cholesterol 33 mg
    Fat 10 g (U)

Grapefruit cocktail
Roast lamb, mint sauce
Broccoli, potatoes
Fruit jelly

    Cholesterol 85 mg
    Fat 10 g (S)

Minestrone soup
Roast chicken
Leeks, potatoes
Apple pie

    Cholesterol 60 mg
    Fat 15.5 g (U/S)

Melon
Risotto (with peas and
    nuts
Ice cream
    Cholesterol 53 mg
    Fat 54 g (U)

French onion soup
Veal cutlet
Cauliflower, potatoes
Fruit yoghurt
    Cholesterol 97 mg
    Fat 40 g (U/S)

Tomato juice
Spaghetti Bolognese
Stewed plums, custard

Cholesterol 81 mg
Fat 23 g (S)

Pineapple juice
Nut and cheese loaf
Sprouts, potatoes
Baked apple with raisins
Cholesterol 21 mg
Fat 17 g (U/S)

Light Meals
Cottage cheese salad
Jam tart

Cholesterol 23 mg
Fat 8 g (U)

Cornish pasty
Coleslaw
Stewed plums
Cholesterol 56 mg
Fat 30 g (U/S)

Rissole
Potatoes
Pear
Cholesterol 54 mg
Fat 26 g (U/S)

Lentil cutlets
Broccoli
Orange
Cholesterol 0
Fat 14 g (U)

Tomato soup
Toast with salmon
 spread
Tinned pineapple
Cholesterol 10 mg
Fat 16 g (U)

Ham and pickles
Baked potato with
 margarine
Pears in red wine
Cholesterol 75 mg
Fat 36 g (S)

Waldarf salad with
mayonnaise
Biscuits and cheese
Cholesterol 10 mg
Fat 20 g (U)

Kipper
Bread and margarine
Stewed fruit
Cholesterol 85 mg
Fat 23 g (U)

Peppers stuffed with
rice
Chocolate cake
Cholesterol 32 mg
Fat 33 g (U)

Cauliflower and tomato
au gratin
Pear conde
Cholesterol 35 mg
Fat 7.5 g (S)

Ploughman's Lunch
(1 oz cheese)
Apple
Cholesterol 29 mg
Fat 31 g (UflS)

Shepherds pie
Fruit sorbet

Cholesterol 54 mg
Fat 12 g (S)

Turkey salad,
French dressing
Banana
Cholesterol 65 mg
Fat 11 g (UflS)

Fish cake
Peas
Jelly
Cholesterol 28 mg
Fat 17 g (U)

Snacks

Beans on toast

> *Cholesterol* 0
> *Fat* 12 g (U)

Biscuits and cottage cheese

> *Cholesterol* 12 mg
> *Fat* 13 g (U)

Salad sandwich

> *Cholesterol* 0
> *Fat* 12 g (U)

Gingerbread
Tea

> *Cholesterol* 2.5 mg
> *Fat* 9 g (U)

Tomato soup, roll
> *Cholesterol* 0
> *Fat* 3 g (U)

Cheese and pickle sandwich
> *Cholesterol* 29 mg
> *Fat* 19 g (UflS)

Bread, margarine and jam
Tea
> Cholesterol 2.5 mg
> *Fat* 12.5 g (U)

Tomatoes on toast with grated cheese
> *Cholesterol* 14 mg
> *Fat* 15 g (U)

Scone, margarine and jam
Tea
> *Cholesterol* 2.5 mg
> *Fat* 15 g (U)

Toasted muffin
> *Cholesterol* 0
> *Fat* 12 g (U)

Sausage roll

>*Cholesterol* 34 mg
>*Fat* 18 g (UflS)

Toasted tomato and
onion sandwich
>*Cholesterol* 0
>*Fat* 12 g (U)

Glass of beer
Crisps

>*Cholesterol* 0
>*Fat* 10 g (U)

Crumpet with honey
Tea
>*Cholesterol* 2.5 mg
>*Fat* 12.5 g (U)

DRINKS

Don't forget to count your drinks — these can add quite a lot of fat and cholesterol to your diet during the course of a day.

	Measure	Cholesterol mg	Fat g
Beer		0	0
Chocolate, all whole milk	1 cup	34	11.5
Chocolate, all skim milk	1 cup	5	3
Chocolate, ½ whole milk, ½ water	1 cup	17	7
Chocolate, ½ skim milk, ½ water	1 cup	2.5	3
Cocoa, all whole milk	1 cup	34	11
Cocoa, all skim milk	1 cup	5	2
Cocoa, ½ whole milk, ½ water	1 cup	17	6
Cocoa, ½ skim milk, ½ water	1 cup	2.5	2
Coffee, black	1 cup	0	0
Coffee, all whole milk	1 cup	34	9
Coffee, all skim milk	1 cup	5	0.5

Coffee, ½ whole milk, ½ water	1 cup	17	4.5
Coffee, ½ skim milk ½ water	1 cup	2.5	0.3
Coffee with cream	1 cup	20	6
Fruit drinks		0	0
Milk	1 glass	40	11
Tea, lemon	1 cup	0	0
Tea with whole milk	1 cup	8	2
Tea with skim milk	1 cup	1	0.2
Wine		0	0